Microsystem Acupuncture

Microsystem Acupuncture

Dr. Jeffrey Carnett

iUniversity Press
San Jose New York Lincoln Shanghai

Microsystem Acupuncture

Published by iUniverse.com, Inc.

For information address:
iUniverse.com, Inc.
5220 S 16th, Ste. 200
Lincoln, NE 68512
www.iuniverse.com

Illustrations By Dorothy Lee

This book does not replace the services of a licensed healthcacre provider
in the diagnosis or treatment of any disease or illness. The information
presented here should not be used for treatment or prevention of disease
without the advice of an acupucnturists or other medical authority.

ISBN: 0-595-14380-6

Printed in the United States of America

Dedication

This book is the culmination of many years of my studies and practice of Chinese Acupuncture. This book has gradually taken form with my feeling that there is a need for a book that provides for a practical method of learning acupuncture and its real life practice.

Along the way many talented doctors of oriental medicine have taught me and given me the incentive to continue my studies and my plans for writing this book. I would like to express my deepest thanks to Dr. John Roberts who provided my first training in Chinese Medicine. His efforts to help me to grasp the concepts and learn what really works have made my work in acupuncture possible.

I would like to also thank Dr. Yu Ping Man who took me under his wing after my studies started in Hong Kong. His high energy and passion for Chinese Medicine rubbed off on me and I cherish his friendship and interest in my professional growth.

Last but not least, my wife and children have provided love and support through the tough times of study, practice and writing. Without their patience none of this would have been made possible.

Jeffrey Carnett, DPM, M.Ac.

Table of Contents

Introduction...xi

List of Abbreviations xiii

Section One :The Nose 1

Section Two:The Eyes 5

Section Three:The Tongue 9

Section Four:Ankle and Wrist 19

Section Five:The Second Metacarpal 25

Section Six:Ren Zhong 29

Section Seven:The Foot 33

Section Eight:Treatment of Common Conditions 39

Conclusions..57

Appendix 59

List of Illustrations

Figure 1: Nose Points 3

Figure 2: Eye Points...6

Figure 3: Traditional Tongue Points...............................11–12

Figure 4: New Tongue Points 17

Figure 5: Upper (Wrist) Points...20

Figure 6: Lower (Ankle) Points 22

Figure 7: Second Metacarpal Points................................26

Figure 8: Ren Zhong Points 32

Figure 9: Plantar Foot Points 34

Introduction

Since the introduction of Chinese Medicine to the West in the 1970's there has been a rapid growth of the profession. Along with it many books on the subject have been written, many translations from the original Chinese but also many by western practitioners.

So many books outline location of acupuncture points and give point prescriptions. While there is always room for another such book I feel the largest area of deficit is in the area of Microsystem Acupuncture. Because of the effectiveness of these methods, alone and with traditional acupuncture I present here perhaps the only comprehensive handbook on the subject.

Microsystem acupuncture is a broad category covering acupuncture of the ear, eye, nose, face, hand and foot to mention a few. Auricular acupuncture being one of more common systems is already written in many sources. The microsystems presented here can be used as the sole modality but are often used usually along with more classical point formulae or local points.

The format of this book is as a simple handbook concentrating on practical use of these methods. My aim is to present in a plain but comprehensive way to allow immediate use and easy reference for practitioners. I have also included a brief introduction to basic Chinese Medical and Acupuncture Channel theory in the appendix for those new to Chinese Medicine.

I thank you for taking the time to pick-up this first edition and welcome suggestions for future editions.

List of Abbreviations

All standard acupuncture points use the point name in Pinyin (Putonghua) and use International Point Nomenclature.

Measurements are standard acupuncture measurements:
One cun = the width of the patient's thumb
One fen = 1/10 of 1 cun

The Nose

Introduction:

The nose system theory of acupuncture holds that all areas of the body are reflected in the nose region. The points correspond to areas of the body and can be used to treat any disorder of that body zone.

The ancient TCM classics *Ling Shu* said "Five Zang organs are in the central nose area and the six Fu organs are on the sides of the nose". Therefore, the nose is subdivided into 20 nasal points. Research has further provided new points in addition to the primary points.

Primary Nose Points:

(see figure 1)

The central nose line runs from the forehead straight to Du 26 (Renzhong/Shuigou). The points for brain, throat lung, heart, liver, spleen and testes/ovary at the tip of the nose. Just to either side of this end point are points for the bladder.

The next "line" of points runs from just below the inner canthus and runs down, slightly diagonally ending near the upper end of the nostrils. This line has points for gallbladder, stomach, small intestine, large intestine and kidney.

The third, or most lateral line starts medial to the inner aspect of the eyebrow and runs in a slightly curved fashion ending at the lateral to the nostril openings. Here we find the points of the ear, thorax, breast, neck /upper back, low back, shoulder/arm, hip, thigh, knee lower leg and toe.

New Points:

These are as follows:

a) "Upper hypertension point" at area of Yintang(extra) between the eyebrows

b) "Lower hypertension point" at the very tip of the nose

c) "Uterus Point" between nostrils superior to Du 26.

The Method:

Usual antisepsis is done using rubbing isopropyl alcohol. Using a small gauge needle the needles are inserted .1–.3 inch obliquely. After piercing the skin, gentle twirling is performed to achieve some tingling sensation and to secure the needle in the point. After arrival of qi needle is retained for 20–30 minutes. One course consists of 10 treatments (daily or on alternate days). If needed, course can be repeated but there should be a 5 day interval between treatment courses.

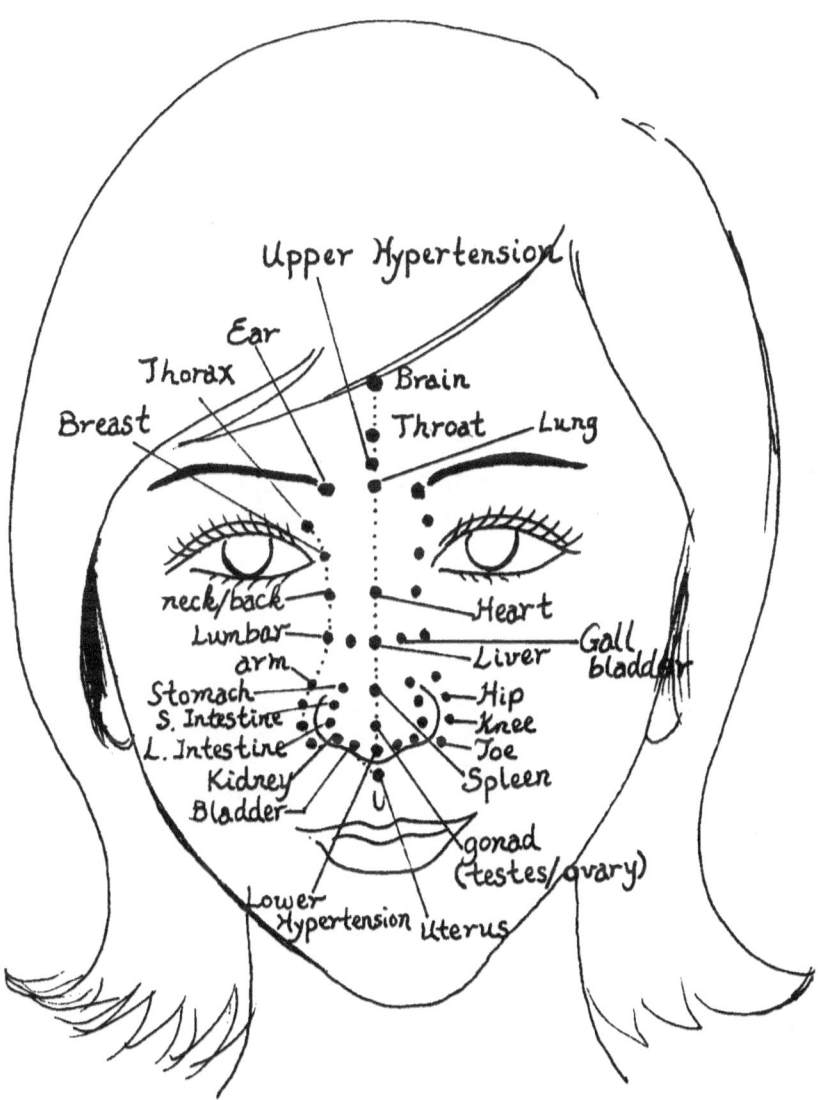

Figure 1

Precautions:

Antisepsis must be used. If you wish, you can use a point finder (fine tipped) but the oils on the nose must be cleaned well with alcohol. After the alcohol is evaporated, then pointer is used. No perpendicular insertion should be used since the tissue of the nose is thin. Avoid puncturing scars. No vigorous manipulation is required nor advised.

Diagnostics:

The corresponding areas of the points might show pain or skin changes. This can be used as diagnostic an indicator that perhaps there is qi imbalance in that region. It is not as evident in the nose as we will see in other systems.

Section Two

The Eyes

Introduction:

Ocular acupuncture is a relatively new therapy credited to Dr. Peng Jingshan. The basic theory was attributed to the ancient famous physical Hua-to. Hua-to commented that physicians should "look at the eyes". Clearly the eyes are mainly used for diagnostic purposes. As an extension of that, the regions of skin around the orbit can be used for therapy.

According to Dr. Peng, the eye is divided into eight regions. He conveniently numbered the regions 1-8. The left eye is numbered clockwise while the right eye is numbered counterclockwise. As follows:

    1 = Lung/Large Intestine

    2 = Kidney/Bladder

    3 = Upper-jiao

    4 = Liver/Gallbladder

    5 = Middle-jiao

    6 = Heart/Small Intestine

    7 = Spleen/Stomach

    8 = Lower-jiao

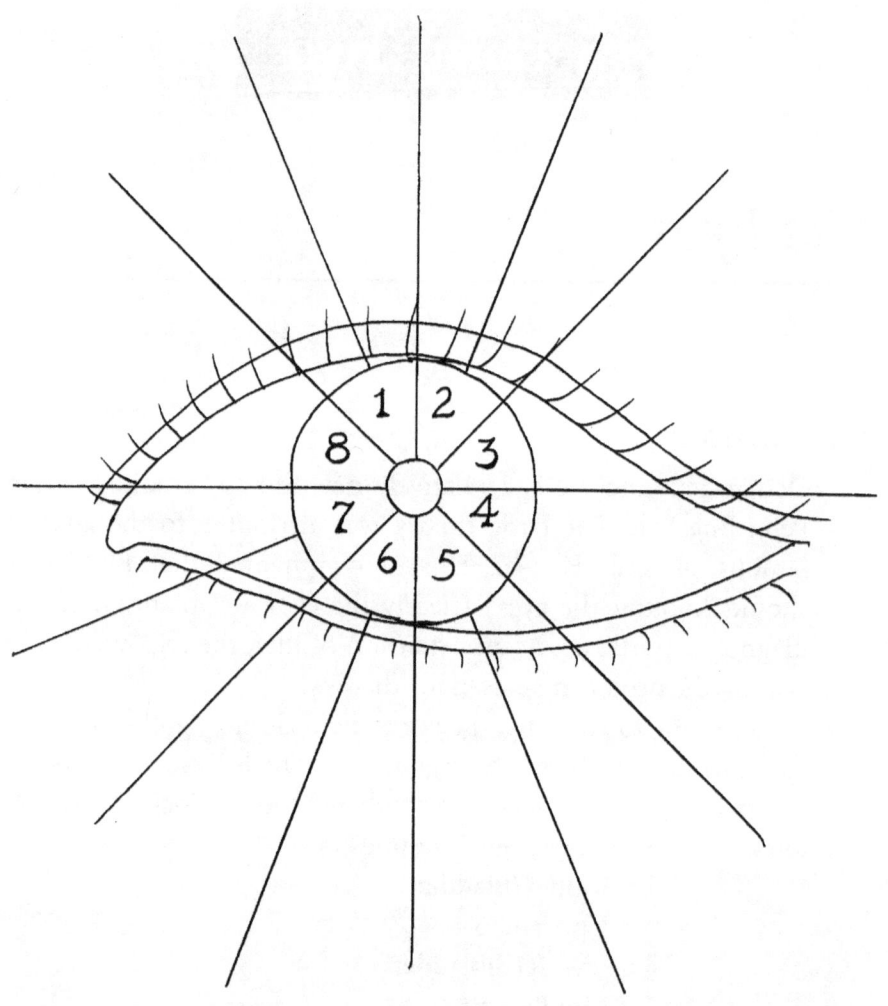

Figure 2

Diagnosis:

With body disorders there can be irregularities or pigmented areas in the sclera of the eye. When these are noticed, they demonstrate imbalances in the corresponding eye region 1-8. For example, a prominent dark blood vessel in region # 4 can be seen with liver qi stagnation or even hemorrhage.

Method:

Points are .2 cun in from the orbit ridge in each of the eye regions.

Strict antisepsis is used. Use fine needles .5cun in length. The needles are inserted against the orbit bone ridge very quickly and shallow, obliquely into the periosteum. No manipulation is used. At insertion there should be a qi arrival sensation. If not, evaluate the point location and repeat needle insertion if needed. Many doctors (including myself) prefer to avoid repeated eye point puncturing at one sitting. The arrival of qi while reassuring might not be that necessary. Needles are retained for 10–25 minutes. On removal apply pressure immediately to decrease chances of bruising.

Microcurrent therapy can be done in this area. Very low insensity uses and perioccular muscle twitching is not desired.

Point Selection:

There are several methods used in determining eye points for treatment.

1) Observe for changes in color, shape of blood vessels in the sclera. If changes are noted, the points are selected in corresponding areas.

2) Use points where there are blood vessel changes when this corresponds with a known diseased area.

3) Select point purely based on known disease location (even with no noted changes in eye blood vessels).

4) Use triple-burner points of eye for treatment of conditions in respective areas. For example, use eye point for upper burner for conditions of the head and face, middle burner point for conditions of the spleen and stomach and lower burner point for lumbo-sacral and lower limb disorders.

5) Point detection method: treat any eye points which are tender to palpation. These points might feel "sore" "numb and cold" or otherwise uncomfortable. Needle these points.

The Tongue

Introduction:

The tongue has been an important organ in Chinese Medicine from ancient times and continues until this day.

In TCM, the tongue is used in diagnosis. It is postulated that the tongue surface is a mirror of the body organs and channels. This can be explained since all organs are connected to the tongue through their channel and collaterals. Let us then take it one step further. If these regions of the tongue reflect the organ conditions, these zones can also be used to influence the condition of the organs. Based on this, Chinese researchers and practitioners has used the following tongue system with consistent therapeutic results.

Method:

The patient should rinse their mouth and gargle with dilute hydrogen peroxide or an antiseptic mouthwash immediately prior to tongue acupuncture.

Points are pierced with fine 30 gauge needles. No twirling needed. Needles retained for 5 seconds then quickly withdraw needle and allow bleeding. After treatment, have patient rinse the mouth again.

Countra-indication: Bleeding disorders/ Anticoagulant therapy.

Tongue Placement for treatment:

Ventral tongue points: The patient opens their mouth and lifts the tongue to gently stabilize against the hard palate near the soft-hard palate border on the roof of the mouth. Points here are pierced to allow slight bleeding.

Dorsal tongue points: Patient opens mouth normally, allows tongue to protrude comfortable with out forcing it out. This will allow tongue to keep normal shape for treatment.

Points:

Traditional Tongue Points:
(see figure 3a & 3b)

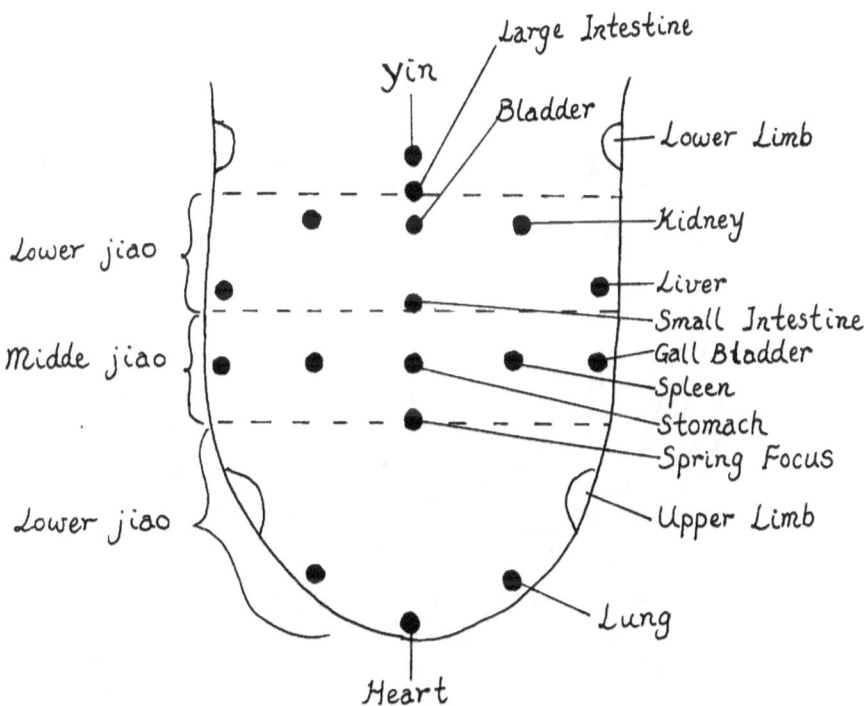

Figure 3a

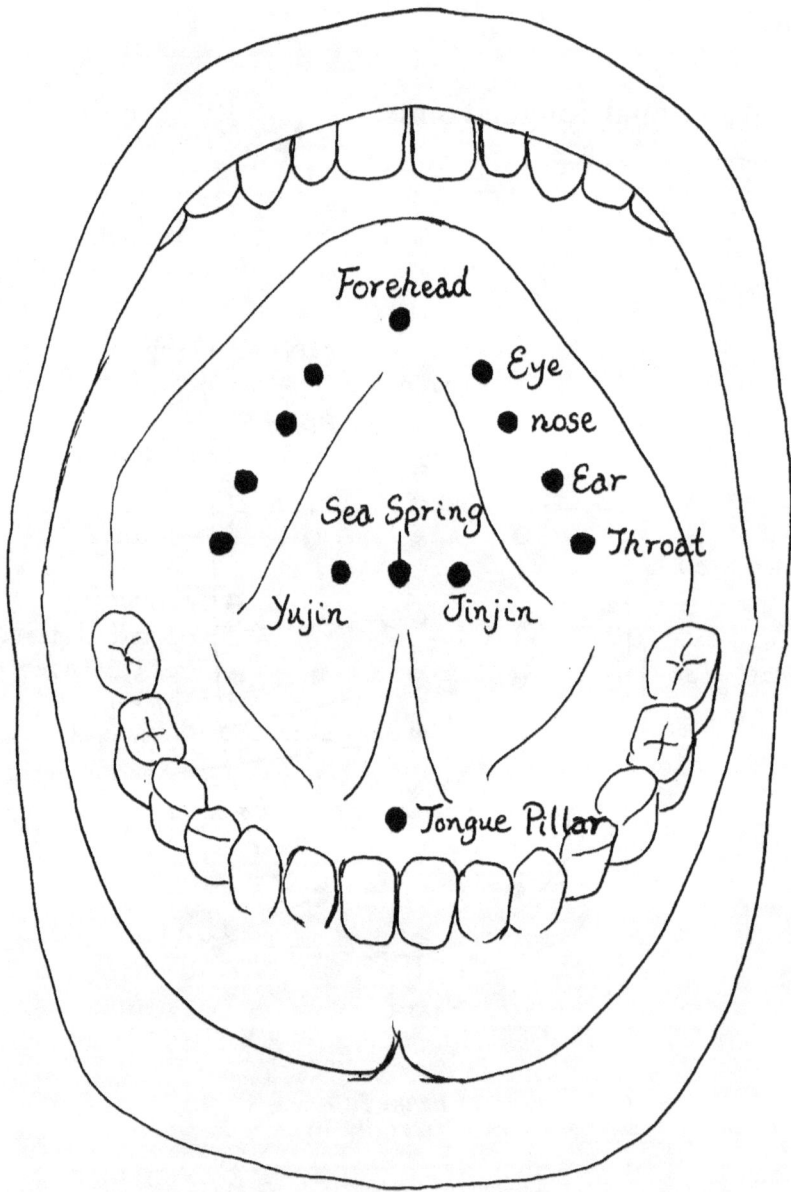

Figure 3b

1) ## Heart Point

   Location: On the dorsal surface of the tongue at the tip.

   Usage: Ant disorder of the Heart Channel.

2) ## Lung Point

   Location: On the dorsal surface of the tongue, paired points 3 fen lateral to the Heart Point.

   Usage: Any Lung Channel Disorder.

3) ## Stomach Point

   Location: On the central dorsal area of the tongue proper. It is 1 cun proximal to the heart point.

   Usage: Any disorder of the Stomach Channel.

4) ## Spleen Point

   Location: These are paired points located 4 fen on either side of the Stomach Point.

   Usage: Spleen Channel disorders.

5) ## Gallbladder Point

   Location: Paired points, 8-fen lateral to the Stomach Point

   Usage: Any Gallbladder Channel disorders.

6) ## Liver Point

   Location: Paired points located 5 fen behind the Gallbladder Points.

   Usage: Liver Channel disorders

7) ## Small Intestine Point

   Location: 3 fen proximal to the Stomach Point on the midline.

   Usage: Any disorder of the Small Intestine Channel.

8) Bladder Point

Location: 3 fen proximal to the Small Intestine Point
Usage: Any Bladder Channel problems.

9) Kidney Point

Location: These are paired points, 4 fen on either side of the Bladder Point.
Usage: Any Kidney Channel disorders.

10) Large Intestine Point

Location: 2 fen proximal to the Bladder Point
Usage: Any Large Intestine Channel disorder.

11) Yin Point

Location: At the root area of the tongue, 2 fen behind the Large Intestine Point.
Usage: Disorders involving the Anus or genitals.

12) Spring Focus Point

Location: In the central area of the tongue proper, 2 fen in front of the Stomach point.
Usage: Resolves excessive thirst and cures tongue stiffness.

13) Upper-limb Point

Location: Between the Lung and Gallbladder Points near the edge of the tongue. This is a paired point.
Usage: Disease and pain of the arms.

14) Lower-limb Point

Location: These are paired points, 1 cun lateral to the Yin Point, near the edge of the tongue.
Usage: Paralysis of the legs.

15) San Jiao Zones

Location: Make a horizontal line through the Spring Focus Point on the dorsal tongue surface. This line is called Line #1. The Area from Line #1 to the tongue tip is the Upper Jiao Zone.

Make a horizontal line through the Small Intestine Point on the tongue surface. This is called Line #2. The area from Line #2 to Line #1 is the Middle Jiao Zone.

Make a horizontal line through the Large Intestine Point on the tongue surface. This is called Line #3. The are between Line #3 and Line #2 is the Lower Jiao Zone.

Usage: These zones are used to aid in differentiation of location of disorders into the Upper, Middle or Lower Jiao. Therefore, mainly diagnostic is usage.

16) Forehead Point

Location: On the bottom of the tongue 3 fen behind the tip.
Usage: Headache and dizziness.

17) Eye Point

Location: On the bottom of the tongue, oblique to the Forehead Point 3 fen. These are paired points.
Usage: Pain and swelling of the eyes.

18) Nose Point

Location: These are paired points located 2 fen behind the Eye points.
Usage: Nasal Congestion or other conditions affecting the nose.

19) **Ear Point**

Location: 2 fen obliquely behind the Nose Points.
Usage: Tinnitus and deafness.

20) **Throat Point**

Location: 2 fen Behind the Ear Point
Usage: Swelling and pain of the throat.

21) **Sea Spring Point**

Location: On the bottom surface of the tongue in the central area just distal to the vertical ridge of skin.
Usage: Resolves excessive thirst.

22) **Jin Jin and Yu Jin**

Location: These are a set of points on the blood vessels on the bottom of the tongue. The blood vessels run on either side of the Sea Spring Point. The Point Jin Jin is the point on the left and Yu Jin the point on the right side.
Usage: To reduce heat as in oral ulcers and chancre sores. Also, inflammation of the tongue and numbness of the throat.

23) **Tongue Pillar**

Location: On the skin flap on the bottom of the tongue at the root area.
Usage: Heavy and swollen tongue.

New Points:
(see figure 4)

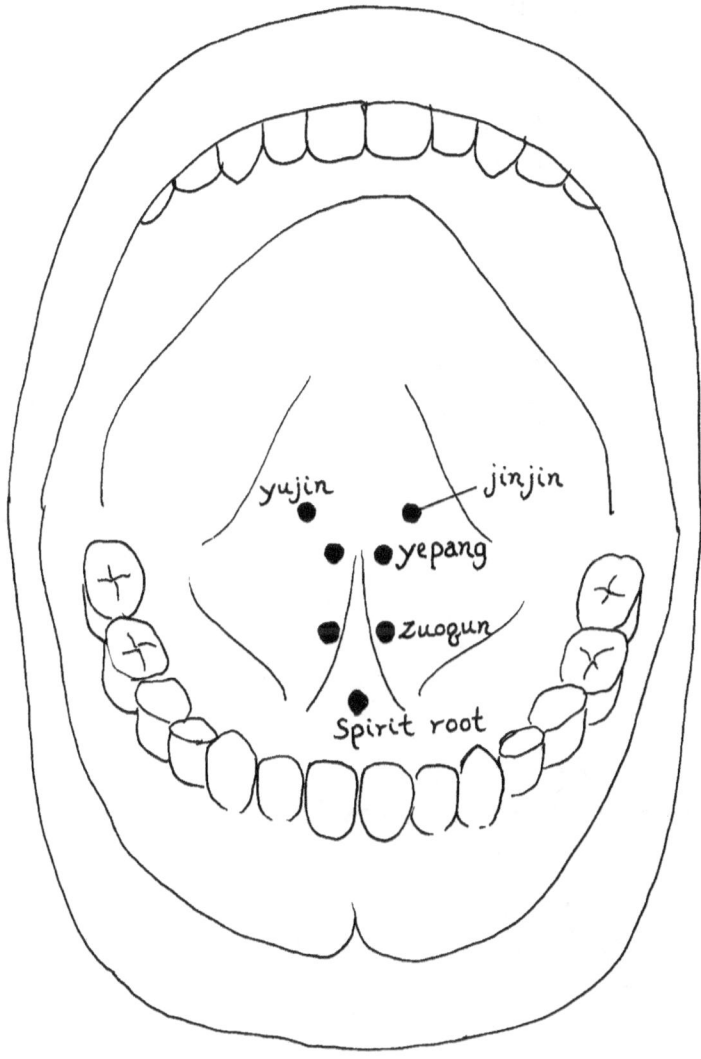

Figure 4

24) Spirit Root Point

Location: On the bottom of the tongue at the root of the tongue. It is at the very proximal aspect of the skin flap.

Usage: Hypertension, cerebral aneurysm.

25) Zuoqun Point

Location: On either side of the flap of skin at the tongue root, midway of the flap length.

Usage: Post Stroke therapy

26) Yepang Point

Location: Paired points oblique to Jin Jin and Yu Jin Point in the proximal 1/3 of the tongue.

Usage: Hypertension and post-stroke.

Ankle and Wrist

Introduction:

The use of needling to the wrist and ankle was developed in modern times in Xi'an, China. There researchers developed the theory that the various sides of the ankle and wrist joints would be linked to specific zones in the body. The technique is simple. No arrival of qi is needed. Simply insert the needle to the hypodermal layer. Some report that less sensation the better the effect.

Wrist Points:

For convenience the points are labeled as follows:
(see figure 5)

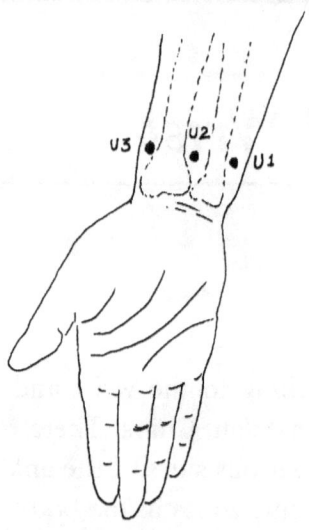

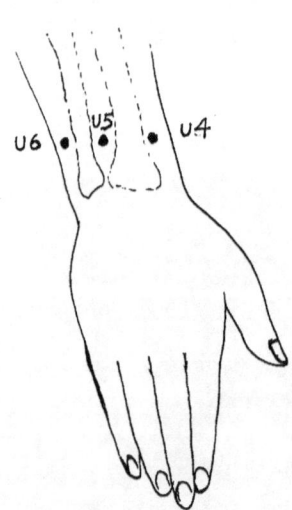

Figure 5

Upper Point #1:

On the palmar aspect of the forearm, between the internal (ulnar) side and flexor ulnaris muscle, 2 cun up from the transverse wrist crease.

Usages: Frontal head pain, eye, nasal problems, facial edema, toothache, bell's palsy, bronchitis, stomachache, cardiac disease, dizziness, hypertension and insomnia.

Upper Point #2:

On the palmar surface of the forearm between the palmaris longus muscle and flexor radialis muscle, 2 cun up from the transverse wrist crease.

Usages: Anterior temple pain, submandibular pain and swelling, asthma, palm pain, numbness of fingertips.

Upper Point #3:

On the palmar forearm, radial to the radial artery, two cun from wrist crease.

Usage: Hypertension and chest pain.

Upper Point #4:

On the dorsal aspect of the forearm, on the radial edge. Two cun above wrist crease.

Usage: Parietal headache, ear problems, Temporal mandibular joint problems, shoulder joint inflammation/pain, chest pain.

Upper Point #5:

At the center of the dorsal wrist between the radius and ulna bone, two cun above the wrist crease.

Usage: Posterior temple headache, shoulder pain, numbness in arms, paralysis of arms, tremble, twitching, elbow pain, wrist and finger pain.

Upper Point #6:

At the lateral border of the ulna, two cun above the wrist crease.

Usage: Occipital headache, head vertex pain, nape of neck pain, chest and upper spinal pain.

Ankle Points:

(see figure 6)

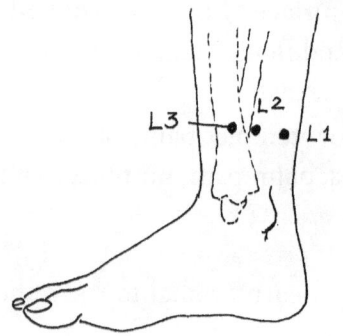

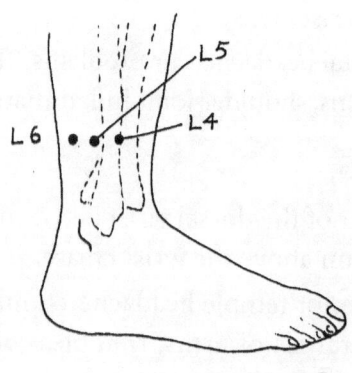

Figure 6

Lower Point #1:

On the anterio-medial aspect of the Achilles tendon 3 cun proximal to the highest point of the medial malleolus.

Usage: Upper abdomen pain and distension pain around the umbilicus, gynecological disorders, enuresis, heel pain.

Lower Point #2:

At the posterior border of the tibia three cun above the highest point of the medial malleolus.

Usage: Allergic type enteritis, lateral abdomen pain.

Lower Point # 3:

One-cm medial to the anterior crest of the tibia, three cun above the highest point of the medial malleolus.

Usage: Medial knee pain.

Lower Point #4:

On the lateral ankle in the area between the anterior border of the fibula and the posterior border of the tibia. 3 cun proximal to the highest point of the lateral malleolus.

Usage: Pain in the knee joint, quadriceps muscle pain, lower limb numbness, tremor, toe pain.

Lower Point #5:

At the posterio-lateral border of the fibula 3 cun proximal to the highest point of the lateral malleolus.

Usage: Hip joint and lateral ankle pain.

Lower Point #6:

AT the lower border of the Achilles tendon (laterally) 3 fingers above the highest point of the lateral malleolus.

Usage: Acute lumbar sprain, sciatica, calf muscle pain.

Method:

Using a 1.5–2 cun long needle. The points are cleaned in the usual skin manner. Using the opposite hand, stabilize the skin of the point to be treated. The needle is inserted quickly at a 30-degree angle away from the foot/hand. The needle should be advanced at the subcutaneous level. This should give no discomfort to the patients. If there is soreness, the needle has been inserted too deeply and should be gently withdrawn to the proper level.

In the use of ankle and wrist points, there is never any manipulation to the needle. Instead, the needle is left at the proper level for about 30 minutes. This treatment is done daily or on alternate days for 10 treatments.

Section Five

The Second Metacarpal

Introduction:

This little known system of acupuncture was first presented by Chinese doctors in the early 1990's. As in other systems already discussed, researchers noticed that there was corresponding pain along this area when certain body parts were in pain, etc.

In this system, the treatments are limited to points along the second metacarpal bone of the hand. All points are along the palmar medial aspect of the bone. The points are as follows (see figure 7):

1) Head Point   Distal

2) Lung Point

3) Liver Point

4) Stomach Point

5) Abdominal Point

6) Waist Point

7) Foot Point   Proximal

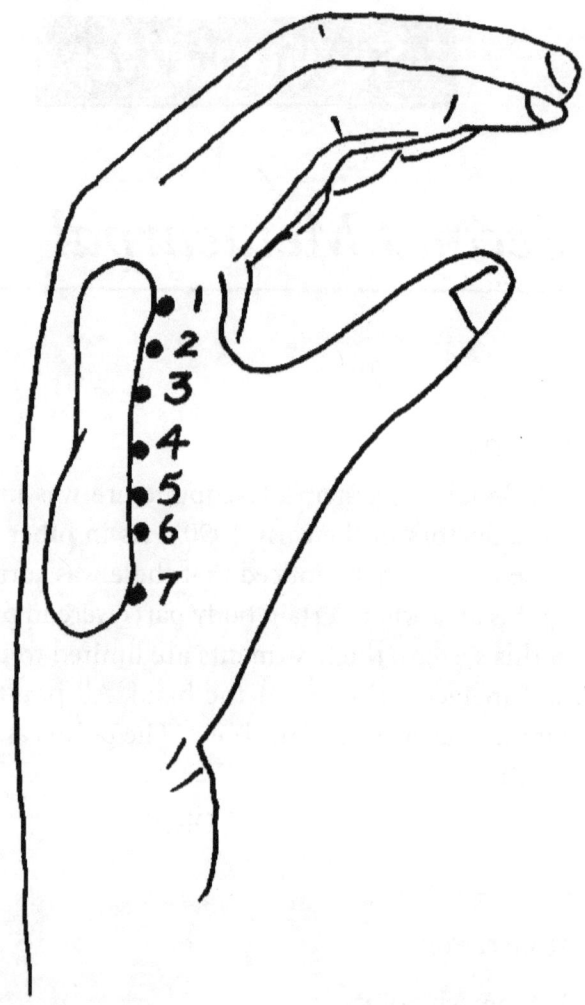

Figure 7

Points:

For convenience of point location points are found based upon the two end points (head and foot) as landmarks.

Head Point:

Located at the distal aspect of the second metacarpal bone on the palmar surface of the head.

Usage: Disorders of the head region, nerve or psychiatric disorders.

Foot Point:

Located at the base of the second metacarpal bone below the base of the bone.

Usage: Disorders of the feet and leg, including cold feet and ankle joint injury.

Stomach Point:

Located at mid-point between the Head and Foot points.

Usage: Gastric disorders such as gastritis and gastric ulceration.

Lung Point:

Located midway between the Head and Stomach Points.

Usage: Any lung or cardiac disorders.

Liver Point:

Located at the mid-point between the Lung and Stomach Points.

Usage: Liver or Gallbladder disorders.

Abdominal Point:

On a line connecting the Stomach and Foot points, this point is at the area 1/3 of the distance down from the Stomach Point.

Usage: Intestinal disorders including diarrhea and constipation or poor digestion. Also benefits all organs not otherwise represented in other points. Lower abdominal pain.

Waist Point:

On a line connecting the Stomach and Foot points, this point is 1/3 of the way up from the Foot Point.

Usage: Kidney, bladder or lower back pain.

Method:

The point to be treated is located by finger pressure and other manual palpation. The area for treatment is usually tender thus suggesting an imbalance in that region. Next, the skin is cleaned in the usual manner. Next, using a 1-1.5 cun needle (30gauge) the point in punctured perpendicularly. The needle is directed to the point, which lies near the periosteum of the second metacarpal bone, about .8 cun deep on average. Once there is strong sensation, the needle is left inplace for 30 minutes. Needle can be gently twirled at 5-10 minute intervals.

Section Six

Ren Zhong

Introduction:

This microsystem is called the "Ren Zong" system. The name comes from the Chinese term for the area of the face between the nose and mouth. In this small area lie 9 individual points used for treatment of groups of conditions.

This area is further divided into 3 segments. These are named Upper, Middle and Lower segments. In each segment there are three individual points (see figure 8).

Nomenclature: Starting from just above the upper lip is the "first" point with the ninth or "last" point just below the nose. These points are named in Chinese "Gou" 1, "Gou" 2, etc.

Here I use the abbreviation "G" with the respective number.

Points:

G1:

Usage: Treatment of conditions affecting the head region such as emergency:

G2:

Usage: Treatment of head, neck and upper back pain, stroke, and facial numbness.

G3:

Treatment of heart and lung, chest (Upper-jiao), back, arm, wrist regions.

G4

Treatment of Chest, upper abdominal, flank area, stomach distension and pain, breast pain, mastitis, etc.

G5:

Treatment of Middle-jiao. That is, spleen, stomach diseases. Also low back pain. This included acute low back strain.

G6:

Treatment of Lower—jiao. That is, kidney, liver and also low back pain.

G7:

Treatment of Liver, kidney diseases and any conditions from the lower abdomen to the knees.

G8:

Treatment of both legs from (and including) knees especially, pain, inflammation and swelling of the legs.

G9:

Used in therapy together with G8 and mainly addresses nasal pain, dry nose, etc.

Summary:

Upper segment (G7,8,9) used mainly for treatment of Lower-jiao, lower limbs, liver, kidney, bladder conditions.

Middle segment points (G4,5,6) are mainly used in treatment of Middle-jiao including stomach, spleen, waist, lower abdomen, etc. conditions.

Lower segment (G1,2,3) are used mainly for Upper-jiao cases including head, nape of neck, upper back, thoracic area, heart and lung conditions.

Method:

The patient should lie down on the treatment table for treatment. The skin is prepared in usual aseptic manner. Next the points are selected based upon condition by channel, Sanjiao or physical location of condition. The point is quickly pierced with a sterile needle to allow two drops of blood to leak from the point. The point is then cleaned with an antiseptic pad.

Contraindications being same as for other bloodletting techniques.

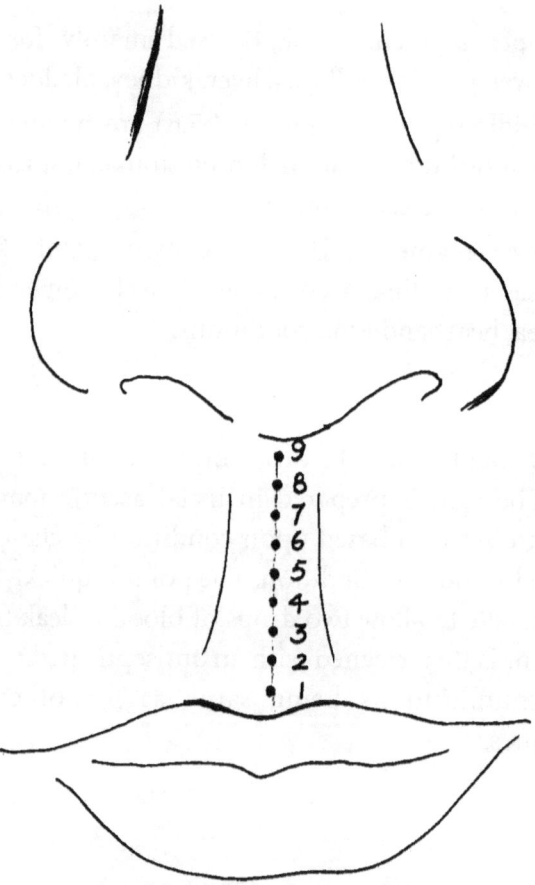

Figure 8

The Foot

Introduction:

Being initially trained as a foot specialist, I entered the field of acupuncture from the foot. At that time I was seeking new modalities that I could use to help my foot patients. I soon found that while acupuncture was very effective in treatment of foot disorders the points on the foot had profound systemic effects.

In Chinese Acupuncture it is theorized that the qi or "energy" of the body is flowing through Channels or Meridians. The classic acupoints lie on these lines. All of the main channels of the body connect in one way or another to the foot. We know that acupuncture treatment is simply a manual excitation of the qi to help the flow in the channels to balance. This being the case, the foot with its pool of channel qi would be an ideal place to perform needling for treatment.

The foot points are numerous and lie on the sole, dorsum as well as medial and lateral aspects of the foot. The field of foot acupuncture can be quite vast so here I will present the most useful points on the sole of the foot. (I hope in future books to discuss the other points as part of a general body acupuncture text-stay tuned.)

The shortcoming of foot acupuncture is that the mere idea of puncturing the sole of the foot with needles makes anyone's skin crawl. However, these treatments are very effective especially in hard to treat cases. Also, with tube needle insertion, the discomfort if very brief. If however the doctor or patient cannot accept this idea, these points can be massaged or stimulated with electrical stimulation (TENS, etc.) I have found that with a little preparation and encouragement patients can accept needle insertion and tolerate it well in general.

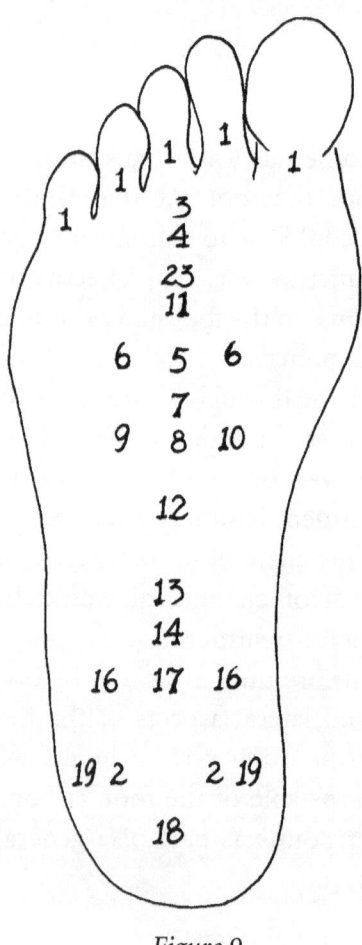

Figure 9

The Points:

Here I present the most commonly used plantar foot points.

1) **EX-PF 1:**

   Location: 5 points on each foot located on the plantar aspect of the proximal interphalangeal joints.

   Usage: Digestive problems, diuretic, loosens local joints.

2) **EX-PF 3:**

   AKA Ear Point

   Location: This point is on the bottom of the heel, 1.5 cum on either side of the mid-point of the heel.

   Usage: Vertigo, tinnitus.

3) **EX-PF 4:**

   AKA Anus Point

   Location: 1 cun posterior to the junction of the 2nd and 3rd toes.

   Usage: Aids in stomach and intestinal function, used in treatment of hemorrhoids.

4) **EX-PF 10:**

   Location: On the bottom of the foot just 1 cun proximal to the 2nd and 3rd toe junction.

   Usage: Stops diarrhea regulates stomach function, diuretic.

5) **Kidney 1:**

   Location: On the bottom of the foot in the middle of the metatarsal arch.

   Usage: This is the starting point of the Kidney Channel so is used for kidney channel disorders like incontinence of urine or stool. It is used for acute problems such as mania, epilepsy, stroke, and coma.

6) **EX-PF 12:**

AKA Kidney Point

Location: 2 paired points 1 cun on either side of Kidney 1.

Usage: Asthma, fever, cough, urine retention, spasms of toes.

7) **EX-PF 13:**

AKA: Stomach Point

Location: On the bottom of the foot 0.5 cun posterior to Kidney 1.

Usage: Stops vomiting, hiccups and overall stomach function.

8) **EX-PF 14**

AKA: Sole Point

Location: On the sole 3 cun posterior to Kidney 1.

Usage: Stomachache, vomiting, indigestion, and foot edema.

9) **EX-PF 15**

AKA: Small Intestine Point

Location: It is on the sole 1 cun on the lateral side of EX-PF 14.

Usage: Stops diarrhea.

10) **EX-PF 17:**

AKA: Liver Point

Location: On the sole of the foot 1.2 cum medial to EX-PF 13.

Usage: Flank pain, sour taste in the mouth, night crying in children.

11) EX-PF 18:

>   AKA: Bladder Point
>   Location: On the bottom of the foot 1 cun distal to Kidney 1.
>   Usage: Foot drop, lumbago, anal prolapse in children.

12) EX-PF 20:

>   AKA: Hypnotic Point
>   Location: .8 posterior to EX-PF 13.
>   Usage: To calm the mind. Used for insomnia, fear, poor memory. Also, heel pain, leg and foot spasm, and paralysis of the lower limb.

13) EX-PF 21:

>   AKA: Heart Point
>   Location: On the sole of the foot 5 cun distal to the middle of the heel.
>   Usage: Calms the mind. Used for hypertension, palpitations of the heart, insomnia from excessive dreaming, tongue inflammation.

14) EX-PF 22:

>   Location: On the bottom of the foot 4.5 cum distal to the middle of the heel.
>   Usage: To improve health overall and stop pain. Used for tumor pain and foot pain.

15) EX-PF 23:

>   AKA: Genital Organ Point
>   Location: On the bottom of the foot .3 cun distal to EX-PF 18.
>   Usage: Impotence, seminal emission, infertility, irregular menstruation, pain in the waist, habitual abortion.

16) **EX-PF 24**

AKA: Leg Point

Location: On the sole of the foot 1 cun lateral to EX-PF 26.

Usage: Leg pain especially "cold" pain in the leg, heel pain.

17) **EX-PF 26:**

AKA: Throat Point

Location: In the midline of the sole, 3.5 cun distal to the middle point of the heel.

Usage: Aphonia, clears throat, laryngitis, tonsillitis.

18) **EX-PF 28:**

AKA: Head Point

Location: On the midline of the sole, 1 cun distal to the posterior border of the heel.

Usage: Headache, fever, stroke, lumbago, swelling and pain in the heel.

19) **EX-PF 29:**

AKA: Eye Point

Location: .6 cun lateral to the midline of the foot, 2 cun distal to the posterior heel edge.

Usage: Headache, vertigo, post-polio syndrome.

Method:

The foot points are cleaned with 70% isopropyl alcohol. Then the needle is placed .1 or .2 cun into the skin. They are left in place for 5-10 minutes. They can also be pricked for bleeding, then bandage applied for 1 hour.

Treatment of Common Conditions

Headache

Eye Points:

Upper-jiao Point, Gallbladder Point for temporal headaches, Bladder Point for Occipital (posterior) headaches.

Nose Points:

Heart Point, Head Point.

Wrist/Ankle Point:

Occipital Headache: Upper #6
Vertex Headache: Upper #4
Frontal Headache: Upper # 1

Second Metacarpal:

Head.

Foot:

EX-PF 28

Trigeminal Neuralgia (Bell's Palsy)

Eye Point:
Upper-jiao Point

Wrist/Ankle Point:
Upper #1

Second Metacarpal:
Head.

Insomnia (with excessive dreaming)

Eye Point:
Upper-jiao Point, Heart Point.

Wrist/Ankle Point:
Upper #1

Second Metacarpal:
Head, Lung, Liver.

Foot:
EX-PF 14, EX-PF 20, EX-PF 21 and EX-PF 12.

Forgetfulness

Eye Points:
Upper-jiao, Heart, Kidney

Second Metacarpal:

Head, Lung.

Foot:

EX-PF 20.

Autonomic Nervous System Dysfunction

Eye:

Upper-jiao, Kidney, Heart.

Nose:

Heart, Kidney, Head

Wrist/Ankle:

Upper #1

Loss of Voice after Stroke

Eye:

Upper-jiao, Heart.

Tongue:

Formula A: Zuoqun, Heart, Kidney.
Formula B: Spirit Base Point, Zuoqun, and Yepang.

Second Metacarpal:

Head.

Foot:

Kidney 1, EX-PF 28.

Dizziness

Eye:
Upper-jiao, Liver.

Wrist/Ankle:
Upper #1, Upper #4

Second Metacarpal:
Head, Lung

Foot:
EX-PF 3

Bronchitis

Eye:
Lung.

Nose:
Lung, Throat, Chest.

Wrist/Ankle:
Upper #1

Asthma

Eye:
Liver.

Tongue:

>Lung, Kidney, Spleen.

Wrist/Ankle:

>Upper #2, Upper #1.

Foot:

>EX-PF 12.

Heart Palpitations

Eye:

>Heart

Tongue;

>Heart

Wrist/Ankle:

>Upper #1, Upper #2.

Foot:

>EX-PF 21

High Blood Pressure

Eye:

>Liver

Nose:

>Hypertension Point. Lower Hypertension Point, Heart, Liver.

Wrist/Ankle:

Upper #1, Upper #3

Low Blood Pressure

Eye:

Liver.

Gall Stones/Cholysystiasis:

Eye:

Gallbladder. Liver

Tongue:

Gallbladder, Liver

Wrist/Ankle:

Lower #1, Lower #4, Lower #5.

Second Metacarpal:

Liver.

Foot:

EX-PF 13

Gastritis

Eye:

Middle-jiao

Nose:

Digestion corner, Stomach, Spleen.

Tongue:

Stomach

Wrist/Ankle:

Lower #1, Lower #2

Second Metacarpal:

Stomach

Foot:

EX-PF 1, EX-PF 4, EX-PF 13, EX-PF 15.

Distended Abdomen

Eye:

Middle-jiao, Stomach, Liver

Nose:

Stomach, Large Intestine, Small Intestine, San-jiao.

Tongue:

Spleen, Stomach, Liver, Large Intestine.

Wrist/Ankle:

Lower #1

Second Metacarpal:

Abdominal Point.

Foot:

EX-PF 13, EX-PF 15, EX-PF 16.

Diarrhea, Lower Abdominal Pain

Eye:

Large Intestine, Lower Jiao.

Wrist/Ankle:

Lower #2

Second Metacarpal:

Abdominal Point

Foot:

EX-PF 15, EX-PF 16.

Constipation

Eye:

Large Intestine.

Tongue:

Large Intestine

Wrist/Ankle:

Lower #2

Foot:

EX-PF 1, EX-PF 4, EX-PF 15, EX-PF 16.

Gastric Ulcer

Eye:
Middle-jiao, Stomach.

Tongue:
Stomach, Liver

Wrist/Ankle:
Lower #1, Lower #2

Second Metacarpal:
Stomach.

Foot:
EX-PF 1, EX-PF 13.

Chronic Appendicitis

Nose:
Appendix, Small Intestine, Large Intestine.

Wrist/Ankle:
Lower #2

Second Metacarpal:
Abdomen

Seminal Emission

Eye:
Lower-jiao

Wrist/Ankle:
Lower #1, Lower #4.

Foot:
EX-PF 23, EX-PF 12.

Sciatica

Eye:
Lower-jiao, Gallbladder.

Wrist/Ankle:
Lower #4, Lower #5

Second Metacarpal:
Low-back.

Foot:
EX-PF 22, EX-PF 24.

Knee Pain

Eye:
Lower-jiao

Wrist/Ankle:

>   Lower #4, Lower #3.

Foot:

>   EX-PF 29.

Heel Pain

Eye:

>   Lower-jiao, Gallbladder.

Wrist/Ankle:

>   Lower #1

Foot:

>   EX-PF 24, EX-PF 28.

Dysmenorrhea

Eye:

>   Lower-jiao

Nose:

>   Front Yin

Wrist/Ankle:

>   Lower #1

Second Metacarpal:

>   Low Back Point.

Foot:

EX-PF 23.

Functional Uterine Bleeding

Eye:

Lower-jiao

Wrist/Ankle:

Lower #1

Foot:

EX-PF 23.

Poor digestion in Children

Wrist/Ankle:

Upper #1

Second Metacarpal:

Stomach

Foot:

EX-PF 1

Nocturnal Enuresis in Children

Eye:

Lower-jiao, Liver, Kidney

Nose:

Heart, Kidney, Front Yin

Wrist/Ankle:

Lower #1

Second Metacarpal:

Low Back Point.

Cataract

Eye:

Liver, Kidney, Lower-jiao.

Wrist/Ankle:

Upper #1

Foot:

EX-PF 29

Tinnitus

Eye:

Liver, Upper-jiao

Wrist/Ankle:

Upper #1, Upper #4

Foot:

EX-PF 3, EX-PF 12

Chronic Otitis Media

Tongue:

Ear, Kidney

Wrist/Ankle:

Upper #1, Upper #4

Vertigo

Eye:

Liver, Upper-jiao

Nose:

Liver, Gallbladder, Lower hypertension point, Heart

Wrist/Ankle:

Upper #1, Upper #4

Foot:

EX-PF 3, EX-PF 28.

Stuffy Nose

Eye:

Upper-jiao, Lung

Nose:

Lung

Ren Zhong:

G1

Wrist/Ankle:

Upper #1, Upper #2

Oral Ulceration/Inflammation

Eye:

Heart

Renzhong:

G1

Tongue:

Heart, Spleen, Jin Jin, Ye Jin

Phalangitis

Eye:

Upper-jiao, Lung

Nose:

Lung, Throat

Wrist/Ankle:

Upper #1

Foot:

EX-PF 26.

Toothache

Eye:
Upper-jiao

Ren Zhong:
G1

Wrist/Ankle:
Upper #1 (front tooth pain). Upper #2 (molar tooth pain).

Common Cold

Eye:
Upper-jiao, Lung

Nose:
Lung, Throat

Wrist/Ankle:
Upper #1

Second Metacarpal:
Lung

Prevention of Common Cold

Nose:
Lung

Wrist/Ankle:

Upper #1

Diabetes Mellitus

Eye:

Upper-jiao, Middle-jiao, Lower-jiao

Tongue:

Sea Spring, Spring Focus

Gout

Eye:

Lower-jiao, Gallbladder

Wrist/Ankle:

Lower #1, Lower #4

Conclusions

I hope that this handbook has given some new and practical information on these unique but useful systems of acupuncture.

While the information is brief and simple, this is partly since there is not a large body of research and clinical experience using these points. As a continuation of this work, I would like to compile individual experiences with any of these techniques and report it in a future publication.

Thank you,

J Carnett
Email: jcar102@yahoo.com

Appendix

An Introduction to Chinese Acupuncture

Chinese Medicine is one of the many systems called "traditional medicine". Others include Aryuveda, Tibetan Medicine and Native American medicine, not to mention only a few. Essentially every primitive culture had their own "system" of dealing with illness". Today many of these systems still exist. Others have disappeared either due to inability to provide the effectiveness of "Western Medicine" but more often due to the overall loss of the native culture by so called civilization. Other systems are experiencing new growth due to people seeking options to modern medicine and all of its costs, side effects and shortcomings. Chinese Medicine is a good example of this phenomenon.

Chinese Medicine developed as a science for diagnosing and treatment human ailments starting about 5000 years ago. It developed over centuries but too lost its influence with colonization and invasion of China by foreign powers and missionaries. China benefited a great deal from Western medicine especially in tacking infectious diseases in China. However, with the poverty of WWII and the civil war China was left in 1949 with little money for medicines. This allowed Chinese Medicine to develop especially in poor areas. The result was an integrated use of Chinese Medicine and Western Medicine.

Chinese Medicine or Traditional Chinese Medicine (TCM) is made up of the following areas:

Herbal Medicine

Acupuncture

Tuina (massage)

Orthopedics (bone setting)

TCM Surgery

Clearly the most prominent systems are those of herbal medicine and acupuncture.

TCM Theory

Remember that Chinese Medicine developed in ancient times. Nothing was known of bacteria, fungi and the like. Nothing was known of hormones or enzymes. All that was known was man in the midst of vast nature.

The ancients felt that disease often can be caused by many factors, internal and external. Simply put external factors of wind, heat, dampness, dryness, and cold caused disease by attaching the body surface. Then, if the body immunity cannot deal with these "pathogens" they would move deeper into the body invading the organs.

Given this brief background, we see that herbs are used to "clear heat" (usually diaphoretic) or "relieve dampness" (usually diuretics). Acupuncture points are also used in this way. Through clinical experience, the ancients found that certain acupuncture points alone and in combination had different effects on the body. Not only of relieving pain but of regulating organ function and blood flow. Many of these effects are being explored but most have not been fully explained.

For us as Westerners and especially doctors to use acupuncture there are two approaches. One is to learn the points and how to puncture them. Next, use a cookbook like approach using point prescriptions based upon a Western diagnosis. This will work often.

The other way is to learn and accept the TCM theory and apply the treatments according to the TCM diagnosis and point functions. This will work better than cookbook approach. In this book I have provided a mixture of the two approaches.

I do wish to here explain the signs and symptoms of the channels so that those not trained in TCM to be able to better understand TCM organ theory.

The main channels are named after organs or areas of the body that they govern. The Heart Channel for example passes down the arm but goes through the Heart so points on this channel are sued often for heart conditions such as chest pain. The heart in TCM is also related to the emotions often so the heart channel points can be used for insomnia and some emotional problems. Below is a brief list of the main channels and the primary symptoms:

Lung Channel:

Signs and symptoms: Shortness of breath, lung conditions, skins and body hair related disorders.

Heart Channel:

Signs and symptoms: Fever in palm of hand, pain in arm or axilla, palpitations, flushed face, chest pain, insomnia.

Pericardium Channel:

Signs and Symptoms: same as for heart.

Large Intestine Channel:

Signs and symptoms: Toothache, neck pain, dry mouth, icteric sclera, runny nose, epistaxis and pain in index finger.

Sanjiao Channel:

Signs and symptoms: Deafness, pharynx edema, excess sweating, and pain in outer canthus of eye. Pain along area from outer ear, shoulder, outer arm and ring finger.

Small Intestine Channel:

Signs and symptoms: Verruca, disturbances of fluid transportation, pain in lower chin and neck, posterior shoulder, elbow and arm pain.

Spleen Channel:

Signs and symptoms: Epigastric pain, abdominal distension, poor appetite, diarrhea, heaviness of body, water retention of body. Fatigue.

Liver Channel:

Signs and symptoms: Lumbago, hypochondriac pain, irritability, sour taste in the mouth, diarrhea with undigested food, inguinal hernia.

Kidney Channel:

Signs and symptoms: Low back pain, enuresis, reproduction, libido disorders, ringing in the ears afternoon fever/flushed feeling.

Stomach Channel:

Signs and symptoms: Nausea, vomiting, epigastric pain, abdominal pain, and excessive borborygmus. Acute febrile disease, oral ulcers, knee pain or swelling, pain in breast region. Pain along anterior lateral leg to second toe.

Gallbladder Channel:

Signs and symptoms: Pain in hypochondriac region, sour taste in mouth, pain along lateral legs.

Bladder Channel:

Signs and symptoms: Posterior headache, tightness in popliteal fossa, calf pain, back pain.

About the Author

Jeffrey Carnett has studied Chinese Medicine and Acupuncture since 1988. He has a doctorate degree in Western Medicine (D.P.M.). He has studied Acupuncture in the USA and China. He holds a Master's degree in Acupuncture.

www.ingramcontent.com/pod-product-compliance
Lightning Source LLC
Chambersburg PA
CBHW031240280526
45784CB00004B/1652